THE NEEDLE-FREE SOLUTION

How Neffy Nasal Spray Is Changing The Face Of Anaphylaxis Treatment, One Spray At A Time, Beyond EpiPen.

Lorinda Innis

Table Of Contents

Introduction

The Anaphylaxis Challenge

Anaphylaxis is one of the medical crises that frightens people more than any other condition, even medical experts. Moments after being exposed to an allergen, a severe allergic response that may be fatal might happen, turning an otherwise ordinary day into a race against time. We are at the nexus of medical knowledge, public health, and human experience as we begin our investigation into anaphylaxis and its management.

A complicated physiological reaction involving many different bodily systems is anaphylaxis. When a trigger occurs, the body's defenses respond to a foreign chemical that most individuals don't know is dangerous. The body experiences a series of symptoms as a result of this overreaction, which may quickly progress from a little discomfort to a serious medical emergency.

The signs and symptoms of anaphylaxis are concerning and diverse. Skin responses like hives, itching, or flushed or pale skin may occur minutes, sometimes even seconds, after being exposed to an allergen. The attack usually affects the respiratory system the most, causing symptoms like wheezing, shortness of breath, or a feeling that your throat is closing. There may also be stomach discomfort, which includes nausea, vomiting, or pain in the abdomen. Anaphylaxis may result in a sudden decrease in blood pressure, which can be very hazardous since it can induce dizziness, fainting, or even shock.

Anaphylaxis may be brought on by a wide variety of highly individualized causes. Several foods (including peanuts, tree nuts, fish, shellfish, eggs, and milk), pharmaceuticals (especially antibiotics and nonsteroidal anti-inflammatory drugs), insect stings, and latex are often identified as contributing factors. Even physical activity or exposure to extreme heat or cold may cause an anaphylactic response in some people. The unpredictable nature of this situation makes preventing and treating anaphylaxis more difficult.

In recent decades, anaphylaxis has become more common, especially in Western nations. The rise in cases has been ascribed to several variables, such as changes in eating patterns, external circumstances, and maybe an excessive focus on personal cleanliness, which might impact the development of the immune system. Whatever the cause, anaphylaxis is now a major public health problem due to the rising number of severe allergic responses.

It is essential to comprehend the processes behind anaphylaxis in order to create efficient preventative and therapeutic approaches. Anaphylaxis is fundamentally a hypersensitivity response mediated by the immune system. Immunoglobulin E (IgE) antibodies are released into the body in response to allergens. These antibodies bind to basophils and mast cells, two types of immunological cells. These sensitized cells quickly unleash a barrage of chemical mediators upon further contact to the allergen, with histamine being one of the main offenders.

The classic signs of anaphylaxis are caused by the release of these chemical mediators. Blood arteries enlarge and become more permeable as a result of histamine, which lowers blood pressure and produces swelling. Additionally, it causes the airways' smooth muscles to constrict, which makes breathing harder. The total inflammatory response is exacerbated by other mediators.

The unpredictable nature of anaphylaxis is one of its most difficult features. Even in the same person who is exposed to the same allergen several times, the intensity of a response might change greatly. The severity of the response may be influenced by a number of variables, including the exposure route, the quantity of allergen, and the person's general health. This unpredictability emphasizes how crucial it is to constantly be ready for a severe response, even in cases when prior exposures only caused minor symptoms.

It is impossible to overestimate the psychological effects of always being at danger for anaphylaxis. Severe allergy sufferers may experience anxiety while engaging in daily activities. Even something as basic as going out to eat or attending a social event may need careful preparation and attention to detail. When their kid has severe allergies, parents are frequently on high alert, always looking out for anything that might endanger their child's safety. The psychological load has the potential to significantly impact mental health and quality of life.

It is crucial to get treatment as soon as possible for anaphylaxis because of its potentially fatal nature. The window of opportunity for a successful intervention is small, frequently measured in minutes as opposed to hours. Treatment delays may have catastrophic outcomes since anaphylactic symptoms can worsen quickly and without warning.

Adrenaline, or epinephrine, is the mainstay of anaphylactic therapy. This potent drug rapidly reverses the symptoms of anaphylaxis by dilating blood vessels, opening airways, and bringing blood pressure back to normal. Usually, an auto-injector is used to provide epinephrine; this is a rapid and simple instrument to use in an emergency.

Due to the need to administer adrenaline quickly, there has been a push to promote accessibility to auto-injectors and public education on their usage. Epinephrine auto-injectors are now widely available in workplaces, public areas, and schools. Several jurisdictions have now established legislation enabling trained non-medical individuals to use these injectors in emergency circumstances.

Obstacles to the use of epinephrine in the treatment of anaphylaxis still exist. Reluctance to give medicine may stem from a variety of factors, including fear of needles, ambiguity over the intensity of symptoms, and worry about possible adverse effects. This hesitancy may have dire repercussions as therapy delays may greatly impair results.

In overcoming some of these obstacles, the creation of substitute epinephrine delivery systems, such the newly authorized nasal spray Neffy, is a major advancement. Such advances may help lower the psychological obstacles to prompt treatment by offering a needle-free alternative, perhaps saving lives in the process.

The treatment of anaphylaxis frequently involves many strategies in addition to epinephrine. Corticosteroids and antihistamines may be used to assist control symptoms, but it's crucial to remember that they shouldn't be used in place of epinephrine and shouldn't be given any later. In extreme situations, supportive treatment may be required, such as oxygen therapy and intravenous fluids.

Additionally, the aftermath of an anaphylactic event has to be closely monitored. There is a chance of a biphasic response, in which symptoms reappear hours after the first episode, even after the original symptoms have subsided. Because of this, people who suffer from anaphylaxis are usually kept under observation in a medical facility for a few hours after their first response.

One of the most important aspects of controlling anaphylactic risk is prevention. The main approach for those with known allergies is to strictly avoid triggers. This might include closely reading food labels, enquiring about ingredients in-depth while eating out, and exercising caution when it comes to any environmental exposures. Complete avoidance isn't always achievable, so keeping an emergency action plan on hand and carrying epinephrine on hand are crucial.

We can now more accurately identify certain allergens and determine the likelihood of severe responses thanks to advancements in allergy diagnostics. While component-resolved diagnostics may provide more precise information on the particular proteins that an individual is sensitive to, skin prick testing and blood tests can assist in identifying allergens. Using this data to create individualized management plans might be beneficial.

Immunotherapy could be a possibility for some people who suffer from severe allergies. In order to progressively reduce sensitivity, this therapy entails exposing the immune system to increasing concentrations of an allergen. Immunotherapy has risks and is not appropriate for everyone, although it has the potential to lessen allergic response severity in some people.

Scientists are always looking for novel approaches to therapy and prevention as the area of anaphylaxis research continues to develop. Research is being done on creating formulations of epinephrine that last longer, examining the possibility of using biologics to alter the immune response, and examining the function of the gut microbiota in the development of allergies.

Fighting anaphylaxis requires a strong emphasis on awareness-raising and education. In addition to teaching patients how to use auto-injectors correctly, healthcare practitioners are essential in helping patients create emergency action plans and informing them about their sensitivities. Broader public awareness is also necessary, however. Being aware of the warning symptoms of anaphylaxis and understanding how to act may save lives for everyone onlooker, teacher, or restaurant employee.

Anaphylaxis affects not only the person but also families, schools, and communities. Food allergy policies and procedures in schools have changed dramatically in recent years, with many establishments enacting stringent rules to make allergic children' learning surroundings safer. In a similar vein, the food sector has enhanced its options for those with dietary restrictions and improved labeling procedures in response to the rising incidence of food allergies.

The more we learn about anaphylaxis, the more equipped we are to control and avoid severe allergic responses. But there are still difficulties. The significance of continuing research and innovation in this sector is highlighted by the rising incidence of allergies, the enduring obstacles to prompt treatment, and the continuous need for improved predicting methods.

The real-life tales that underlie the anaphylactic statistics serve as potent warnings of the risks. Anaphylaxis is more than just a medical condition—it's a profound life experience for everyone who has ever faced the terrifying prospect of a severe allergic reaction, for parents who have lived in constant fear of their child's next exposure, and for medical professionals who have sprinted to save a life.

We bring these memories and the optimism that comes from medical progress with us as we continue to investigate anaphylaxis and its treatment. The approval of novel therapies such as Neffy is a sign of optimism for those with severe allergies as well as a scientific accomplishment. It is evidence of the power of creativity motivated by genuine human needs.

Anaphylaxis is a complex problem with medical, psychological, and social aspects. It needs an all-encompassing strategy that incorporates state-of-the-art research, useful solutions, and compassionate care. We are getting closer to a day where the danger of anaphylaxis won't be as great as it once was as we continue to simplify the immune system and create better therapies.

But much as we applaud advancements, we still need to exercise caution. Because anaphylaxis is unexpected, one must always be prepared and dedicate oneself to continuing education and awareness campaigns. Every person who knows about anaphylaxis, every person who carries an auto-injector, and every novel therapy that is created advances our understanding of this difficult medical problem.

In many ways, the story of anaphylaxis is a microcosm of larger themes in contemporary medicine, such as the interaction between environmental factors and genetic predisposition, the necessity of quick action in an emergency, the possibility that treatment barriers will be broken down by technology, and the ability of patient advocacy to effect change.

At this point in time, when novel therapies are being developed and our knowledge of allergy processes is expanding, we are motivated by both optimism and resolve. Despite the difficulty of anaphylaxis, we are prepared to meet it with knowledge, creativity, and a common goal of preserving health and saving lives.

Chapter One

The Evolution of Epinephrine Delivery

The introduction of epinephrine is a tale of continuous innovation propelled by an urgent medical need. For many years, the primary state of emergency care for anaphylaxis, a severe and sometimes fatal allergic response, has been the prompt injection of epinephrine. The development of sophisticated delivery methods from the first crude injections to the present day demonstrates not just technical advancements but also a greater comprehension of patient requirements and the vital significance of prompt, efficient therapy.

In the early days of managing anaphylaxis, the conventional syringe and vial approach was usually used to deliver epinephrine. Even though this method was novel at the time, it had some drawbacks. In an emergency, medical personnel had to draw the right dosage under pressure, which is a laborious and error-prone technique. Due to the intricacy of this procedure, patients or caregivers trying to self-administer often experienced delays or errors that might have serious repercussions.

An important turning point in the treatment of allergy emergencies was the invention of the first epinephrine auto injector in the 1980s. These gadgets, which were best represented by the EpiPen, transformed the industry by offering an easily accessed, pre-measured dosage of adrenaline. The syringe-and-vial method had many drawbacks that were solved by the creation of the autoinjector. It greatly decreased the possibility of user mistake, did away with the need for dosage measurement, and drastically shortened the administration time.

The advantages of conventional autoinjectors were profound and readily noticeable. They democratized the administration of emergency epinephrine, first and foremost. Treating anaphylaxis was no longer limited to medical experts or anyone with specific expertise. With only a little guidance, patients, family members, educators, and other caregivers could now dispense life-saving medicine. Public health was significantly impacted by this change, especially in places like camps, schools, and other community centers where medical assistance may not always be readily accessible.

Furthermore, many allergy patients and their families experienced some psychological relief because of the autoinjector design. They felt secure and in control of their situation knowing they had a little, practical instrument to stave off a serious allergic response. Many people with severe allergies were able to live more normal, active lives because they felt more at ease knowing they had a solid safety net against the worst-case situation.

In an emergency, the autoinjector accelerated the supply of adrenaline. The difference between struggling with a syringe and just removing a cap and pushing a button might be life-altering in anaphylaxis, when every second counts. Research has repeatedly shown that quicker epinephrine delivery is associated with improved anaphylactic episode outcomes.

But like every medical device, the conventional autoinjector format has limits and downsides that were discovered with time and extensive usage. The learning curve for appropriate usage has proven to be one of the biggest problems. Autoinjectors still need some familiarization and training, even if they are more straightforward than syringes. Users have been known to make errors under pressure, such as injecting into the incorrect area of the body or not holding the device in place long enough to administer the medication completely.

One additional noteworthy disadvantage has been the needle-phobia. Even when faced with a severe allergic response, many people—children in particular—find the idea of self-administering an injection to be quite frightening. Due to their needle fear, some patients have been known to hesitate or stop using their autoinjectors completely, endangering their lives needlessly. One of the ongoing challenges in enabling the early and broad administration of epinephrine in emergencies is the psychological barrier posed by the needle.

Traditional autoinjectors have also raised concerns about physical pain. It may take a lot of power to pierce the skin and inject the drug, which often causes discomfort there. Even though this pain is a little price to pay for a life-saving procedure, many patients have expressed worry about it, and in some situations, it has prevented early usage.

Autoinjector mobility and compactness have also posed practical difficulties. Many patients find the devices heavy and cumbersome to regularly carry, particularly in the warmer months when there may be fewer alternatives for clothes. Since the most effective autoinjector is the one that is actually with the patient when anaphylaxis begins, this portability problem has practical ramifications.

In recent years, accessibility and cost have become major disadvantages. Certain name-brand autoinjectors have become very expensive, burdening patients and healthcare systems financially. Due to the economic barrier, people are finding themselves in circumstances where they are either going without or rationing their autoinjector, which goes against medical recommendations for those who are at risk of anaphylaxis.

Traditional autoinjectors have also drawn criticism for their environmental effects. Since the gadgets are usually single-use, a large quantity of plastic and medical waste are produced. This element of autoinjector usage has drawn attention in an era when environmental concern is growing.

Finally, an ongoing problem with autoinjectors has been the duration of the epinephrine's shelf life. Since many patients take their devices with them in a variety of environmental settings, the drug's potential for degradation over time—particularly when exposed to heat or light—is a cause for worry. Because of the comparatively short shelf life, replacements must be made often, which raises the total cost and sometimes results in patients being caught in an emergency with expired medicine.

While these shortcomings of conventional autoinjectors do not diminish their tremendous worth in treating anaphylaxis, they have prompted a quest for substitutes. Pharmaceutical firms, regulatory agencies, and the medical community have acknowledged the need for epinephrine delivery methods that overcome these drawbacks and preserve or even enhance the advantages of autoinjectors.

A comprehensive awareness of patient requirements and public health imperatives is the driving force behind the search for alternatives. Fundamental to it is the understanding that the perfect epinephrine administration method should be readily accessible, simple to administer under pressure, physically pleasant, psychologically acceptable, and medically successful.

Developing the autoinjector design itself has been one avenue of innovation. Aims have been set on producing more manageable, compact gadgets that are simpler to take about on a regular basis. In order to decrease discomfort and accelerate the administration of epinephrine, several more recent versions have concentrated on enhancing the injection process. Others have focused on resolving issues related to cost and dependability by increasing the medication's shelf life inside the apparatus.

Investigating delivery methods that are completely needle-free has been one more development path. This method specifically addresses the problem of needle fear, which has prevented many patients from using epinephrine on time. In this regard, technologies like jet injectors, which use high pressure to push medicine through the skin without the need for a needle, have shown promise.

Although the idea of administering adrenaline orally has also been considered, there are a number of obstacles to overcome, including the fact that adrenaline degrades quickly in the digestive tract and that emergency conditions call for fast absorption. Nevertheless, because of the possible advantages of a really non-invasive delivery technique, research in this field is going.

Epinephrine patches have also been studied; these would gradually apply the drug via the skin. Although unsuitable for the prompt administration required in cases of severe anaphylaxis, this kind of device could provide continuous protection to those who are very susceptible to allergic responses.

Possibly the most promising substitute to emerge in the last several years is the creation of epinephrine nasal sprays. Comparing this method to conventional autoinjectors, there are a number of possible benefits. It gets rid of the necessity for injections, which helps with needle anxiety and the discomfort of intramuscular administration. Under general, nasal sprays are simpler to apply, requiring less instruction and lowering the possibility of user error under stressful circumstances. Due to the nasal mucosa's superior surface for drug absorption, they also provide the possibility of more reliable and quick epinephrine absorption.

The first nasal spray epinephrine medication for anaphylaxis, Neffy, was approved by the FDA, marking a critical turning point in this history. Neffy and related nasal spray technologies might provide equivalent or even better effectiveness in treating anaphylaxis while directly addressing several of the disadvantages of conventional autoinjectors.

Developing innovative devices or delivery systems is not the only step in the process of developing alternatives to conventional autoinjectors. It's a component of a more significant change in the way we handle allergy emergencies. The increasing focus on patient-centered design in medical technology is reflected in this trend. It recognizes that medicines that patients will really employ when necessary—rather than only those that function well in carefully monitored clinical settings—are the most successful.

The need for alternatives also emphasizes how crucial choice is when it comes to medical care. Individual patients possess distinct requirements, inclinations, and situations. The medical community can better serve the broad demographic of patients who are at risk for anaphylaxis by creating a variety of epinephrine administration alternatives.

The development of epinephrine delivery systems also touches on broader themes in healthcare, such the shift to more individualized treatment and the growing importance of patient self-management. Patients are becoming increasingly empowered to manage their allergies on their own terms by selecting the epinephrine administration route that best suits their requirements and lifestyle as new choices for the drug are developed.

The area of epinephrine administration is probably going to keep changing in the future. It's possible that we'll see improvements made to nasal spray technology, fresh ideas for increasing the duration of epinephrine's shelf life, or even brand-new, unimagined delivery systems. Future breakthroughs will be shaped in large part by the continuing conversations that occur between patients, healthcare professionals, researchers, and regulatory agencies.

It's good to take stock of our progress as we think about the future of epinephrine administration. Every step we've taken toward realizing the goal of safe, efficient, and widely available anaphylactic therapy for everyone in need—from the days of bulky syringes to the current selection of autoinjectors and cutting-edge substitutes like nasal sprays—has gotten us closer to that ideal.

In many respects, the history of epinephrine distribution serves as a microcosm of overall medical advancement. It demonstrates how early discoveries may transform healthcare while also posing new difficulties. It highlights the value of taking into account a treatment's accessibility and practicality in addition to its medicinal effectiveness, as well as the usefulness of patient input to spur innovation.

The objective remains unchanged as we proceed: to guarantee that everyone who is susceptible to anaphylaxis has access to epinephrine in a way that allows them to administer it efficiently, swiftly, and with confidence when it counts most. Not only is the transition from conventional autoinjectors to a wide range of delivery methods technologically advanced, but it also aims to save lives and enhance the quality of life for millions of individuals who suffer from severe allergies.

The development of epinephrine delivery methods serves as a reminder that, in the field of medicine, there is always a need for patient education and adaptation. We take the lessons from every iteration into account as we continue to improve and broaden our approaches to emergency allergy care, constantly aiming for greater results and more accessibility to medications that may save lives.

Chapter Two

Introducing Neffy: A Breath of Fresh Air

A novel breakthrough in allergy therapy has surfaced, which has the potential to revolutionize our understanding of severe allergic responses. Neffy, the first FDA-approved nasal spray epinephrine medication for anaphylaxis, is this invention. With Neffy, emergency allergy treatment has advanced significantly as a needle-free substitute for conventional autoinjectors like EpiPen.

The most effective way to treat anaphylaxis is with epinephrine, which is found in Neffy, a nasal spray. This ground-breaking device, created by ARS Pharmaceuticals, attempts to overcome some of the main obstacles connected to conventional epinephrine administration techniques. Neffy's primary function is to quickly and effectively treat severe allergic responses without the need for a needle, which makes it a desirable choice for those who are afraid of injections or find using autoinjectors difficult.

Neffy has a very powerful but beautifully simple idea. Because epinephrine is administered by nasal spray rather than injection, there may be less hesitancy in emergency circumstances. This is especially important since in anaphylactic instances, quick epinephrine delivery may save lives. Since Neffy employs the same spray mechanism as Narcan, the popular naloxone nasal spray for opioid overdose, many people are acquainted with the Neffy nasal spray style.

Neffy works by using the body's own natural channels for absorption. When epinephrine is sprayed into a nose, it quickly enters the bloodstream via the nasal mucosa. This method of administration enables the drug to be quickly distributed throughout the body, which is essential for the urgent treatment of anaphylaxis. A precise amount of epinephrine is delivered via the nasal spray, which is calibrated to provide therapeutic levels that are similar to those obtained with injectable versions.

Neffy's intuitive design is one of its main benefits. Like conventional autoinjectors, the gadget is lightweight, carry-anywhere, and portable. On the other hand, many users could find it less scary since it doesn't need needles. Not only is this simplicity of use convenient, but in the high-stress situation of an allergic response, a less complicated delivery system can be the difference between receiving medicine on time and riskily delaying it.

To guarantee Neffy's effectiveness and safety throughout development, a great deal of research and clinical testing were conducted. Research carried out by ARS Pharmaceuticals revealed that Neffy was able to get blood epinephrine concentrations that were equivalent to those obtained after injection. In addition to further study on children weighing more than 66 pounds, these trials included 175 healthy adults. Similar increases in heart rate and blood pressure, two important markers of epinephrine's physiological effects, were seen in the data.

Resolving FDA concerns over repeat dosage was a crucial part of Neffy's development. Similar to injectable epinephrine, Neffy is designed to enable a second dosage if required. To guarantee the security and effectiveness of this strategy, the FDA did, however, request further information. This is a reflection of the strict guidelines that are applied to novel medicine formulations, particularly for vital emergency drugs.

Neffy's FDA clearance procedure was extensive and included several steps. It required assessing the drug's pharmacodynamics and pharmacokinetics as well as taking public health implications into account. The FDA acknowledged that Neffy might lower obstacles to prompt anaphylaxis therapy, especially for those who would put off or forgo treatment because they are afraid of needles.

The FDA took into account a number of important aspects throughout the approval procedure. These included the medication's safety profile, ability to enhance treatment adherence, and ability to administer epinephrine at the right doses quickly in an emergency. The usability of the gadget was also assessed by the agency, which was crucial considering the important nature of its intended application.

Neffy's FDA clearance procedure was unique in that it included "passerby" investigations. The FDA sought these investigations, which entailed evaluating the product on people who were unaware of Neffy or the therapy for anaphylaxis. The participants were put in emergency situations that were mimicked, such a restaurant where one of the customers was having a severe allergic reaction. After that, they were instructed to read the instructions and provide the medication. With no previous training or guidance, 100% of participants were able to use the gadget properly, which produced outstanding results. This illustrates how Neffy may be useful for onlookers in public places as well as allergy sufferers and their carers.

Neffy was approved by the FDA with certain suggestions and criteria. Adults and children above the weight of sixty-six pounds are permitted to use it; the recommended dose is one spray each nostril. Similar to injectable epinephrine, the approval also contained options for a second dosage if necessary. But after using Neffy, the FDA stressed how crucial it is to get emergency medical attention, stressing that this is a first-line therapy and should not be used in place of professional medical care.

Neffy approved it, but she gave it some serious thought because of its possible shortcomings. According to the FDA, those who have had nasal surgery, have polyps in their noses, or have extreme congestion may find it difficult to absorb the medicine. This emphasizes the need for tailored medical guidance as well as the ongoing significance of injectable epinephrine for some individuals.

Another important factor in Neffy's clearance was its side effect profile. Frequently reported adverse effects include jitteriness, headache, tingling nose, throat irritation, and nasal pain. Given that the medication has the ability to save lives in cases of anaphylaxis, these side effects were judged to be tolerable and mostly in line with the established pharmacological properties of epinephrine.

The clearance of Neffy not only creates new opportunities for research and development but also represents a major turning point in the treatment of allergies. The FDA will likely approve ARS Pharmaceuticals' application for use in younger children, particularly those who weigh between 33 and 66 pounds. This extension may increase the effect of this novel therapeutic strategy.

Neffy's promise goes beyond its immediate use in allergy therapy. The approval of this medicine might lead to the development of alternative needle-free emergency treatments, which could completely change the way we treat a range of acute medical illnesses. Neffy's FDA clearance and clinical trial results show that nasal spray formulations are a viable means of quickly and efficiently administering essential drugs.

From the standpoint of public health, Neffy might have a big influence on how anaphylaxis is treated. It may raise the possibility of administering adrenaline in an emergency circumstance on time by offering a less frightening and simpler substitute for autoinjectors. This may have a special effect in places like restaurants, schools, and airports where non-medical staff may need to handle an allergic response.

Neffy's creation and approval serve as further evidence of the pharmaceutical industry's continuous innovation, especially with regard to medication delivery methods. It is an example of how reevaluating how an existing drug is administered might result in potentially life-saving innovations. This strategy, which takes a well-known medication like epinephrine and finds a creative, more user-friendly manner to distribute it, may be used as a template for similar approaches in the future.

Neffy's real-world performance will be widely watched once it hits the market. Its safety profile and efficacy in a range of groups and situations will be further determined by post-marketing monitoring. As is customary with new drugs, this continuous assessment will provide important information that will inform future recommendations and possible increases in the drug's usage.

Another crucial component of Neffy's market debut is its pricing approach. According to ARS Pharmaceuticals, insurance companies will pay a similar amount for these autoinjectors as they do now, and patient affordability will be guaranteed via established initiatives. By making Neffy available to a larger group of patients, this strategy hopes to boost its uptake and influence.

Neffy's introduction also calls into question the training and education of patients. Despite the device's easy design, it will be important to make sure patients, caregivers, and maybe the general public know how to use it properly. This might include fresh approaches to teaching and training for the general public as well as healthcare professionals.

The allergy community has reacted enthusiastically to Neffy's approval. Numerous professionals consider it a revolutionary advancement that has the potential to save lives by decreasing reluctance to provide adrenaline. It's an intriguing possibility that Neffy may be available in public spaces, much like automated external defibrillators (AEDs), which might enhance the emergency response to anaphylaxis.

Neffy's availability will probably force emergency strategies for anaphylaxis in a variety of contexts to be reevaluated. It could be necessary to amend emergency response plans and procedures at places of employment, public spaces, and schools to include this new treatment option. This may spark more extensive conversations about disaster preparation and allergy awareness in public areas.

Neffy's achievement in receiving FDA clearance also acts as a catalyst for more advancements in the management and treatment of allergies. It indicates that major progress in our approach to even well-established medical problems is possible. This might lead to further research and development in fields including developing new therapies for various allergic disorders, preventing allergies, and developing better diagnostic tools.

Researcher and healthcare provider interest will be piqued in the long-term effects of Neffy on anaphylactic outcomes. Research monitoring Neffy's practical use, including how it affects treatment rates, administration time, and patient outcomes, will provide important light on how successful the program is as a public health measure.

Neffy's creation and acceptance provide more evidence of the value of patient-centered design in medical advancements. Neffy serves as an excellent example of how taking into account patient experiences and preferences may result in substantial breakthroughs in healthcare by removing a major barrier to treatment: the fear of needles.

Neffy may impact our understanding of emergency drug design in general as it is included into allergy management procedures. The success of a nasal spray form for a vital emergency drug may spur the development of other strategies for other ailments where prompt drug delivery is essential.

Neffy's development and approval story is also an example of how medical innovation is collaborative. It featured contributions from patients, healthcare providers, and regulatory agencies in addition to the work of academics and pharmaceutical developers. The successful development of revolutionary medical technology from idea to market often depends on this cooperative approach.

Neffy is a major development in the anaphylaxis therapy field. It's a welcome addition to the toolkit for treating severe allergic responses because of its needle-free design, convenience of administration, and ability to lower obstacles to prompt treatment. With increased accessibility and use, Neffy has the potential to revolutionize the way we handle anaphylactic treatment, perhaps rescuing lives and offering comfort to millions of individuals impacted by severe allergies. The process from conception to FDA clearance highlights the constant advancements in medical research and the never-ending pursuit of better patient outcomes and treatment in life-threatening circumstances.

Chapter Three

The Science Behind Neffy

The creation of Neffy signifies a noteworthy advancement in the management of anaphylaxis. To guarantee its safety and effectiveness, this novel epinephrine nasal spray formulation has undergone extensive scientific testing. From idea to FDA approval, the process involves a great deal of study, careful clinical trials, and in-depth comparisons with other injectable epinephrine choices.

A number of carefully planned clinical trials meant to prove Neffy's effectiveness in quickly and consistently supplying epinephrine to the bloodstream served as the cornerstone of its development. The comparison of Neffy's pharmacokinetics and pharmacodynamics with those of conventional injectable epinephrine was the main goal of this research.

175 healthy people who were carefully chosen to represent a varied cross-section of the population participated in one of the major studies. The purpose of this research was to determine the blood levels of epinephrine after Neffy administration and compare them to the levels obtained with injections of the drug.

The optimistic findings demonstrated that Neffy supplied circulatory levels of epinephrine that were similar. This was an important discovery since it showed that the nasal spray may be just as effective as the most effective injectable type.

Important physiological reactions to epinephrine injection were also investigated in this research. Researchers kept an eye on variations in heart rate and blood pressure, two vital markers of epinephrine's systemic effects. Neffy once again showed increases in these measures that were comparable to those of injectable epinephrine, indicating that it may be a good substitute.

Based on these results, scientists expanded their study to include kids who weighed more than 66 pounds. Given that children make up a significant fraction of the population at risk for severe allergic responses, this pediatric research was crucial. The outcomes were similar to what was seen in adults, with similar blood levels of adrenaline attained. Neffy's potential wide application was strongly shown by its consistency across age groups.

Examining Neffy's commencement of action was one of the clinical study' most interesting features. Every second matters in anaphylaxis, therefore getting epinephrine to the patient quickly is essential. According to the trials, Neffy may quickly reach therapeutic blood levels of epinephrine, similar to the quick effects of injectable versions, in only a few minutes of treatment. In emergency settings, when timely treatment might mean the difference between life and death, this rapid onset is crucial.

Neffy's effectiveness was assessed in terms of both its pharmacokinetic properties and its capacity to mitigate anaphylactic symptoms. Researchers evaluated Neffy's potential efficacy in real-world circumstances using surrogate endpoints and extrapolation from the pharmacokinetic data, despite ethical concerns that prohibit creating severe allergic responses in trial participants. The findings indicated that Neffy might successfully treat the potentially fatal symptoms of anaphylaxis, including tissue swelling, hypotension, and constricted airways.

Researchers were careful to include a few important criteria when comparing Neffy with injectable epinephrine. The primary concern was the difference in epinephrine's bioavailability between nasal and intramuscular injection routes. The investigations revealed that while there were minor variations in the absorption patterns—nasal administration exhibited a more steady increase in blood levels as opposed to an abrupt peak seen with injection—the overall bioavailability was similar. This discovery was essential to proving that Neffy was a good substitute for injections.

The dosage uniformity was another significant contrast. Although injectable epinephrine is effective, its absorption rates might vary based on injection location and method, among other things. Neffy's nasal administration resulted in more uniform absorption patterns across the subjects. In real-world emergency scenarios, when stress and hurry may impair the administration of injectable forms, this consistency may translate into more dependable dosage.

One important consideration when comparing Neffy with injectable epinephrine was how simple it was to administer. Researchers measured participants' nasal spray administration speed and accuracy in comparison to auto-injector use. The nasal spray was far simpler to apply for many participants, particularly for those who had no previous instruction, according to the startling findings. Because it's so simple to administer, it may facilitate quicker administration in an emergency and might raise the possibility that onlookers will provide assistance in the event of an anaphylactic crisis.

Researchers also looked at the possibility of repeat dosage, which is important to take into account when anaphylaxis is severe and a single dose may not be enough. Neffy, like injectable epinephrine, might be safely given in several doses if necessary, according to the research. This discovery was crucial in proving that Neffy was a complete substitute for injections, able to manage the worst allergic responses.

The comparative tests also examined the drug's stability in different scenarios. The effectiveness of epinephrine auto-injectors may be impacted by their sensitivity to temperature extremes. Neffy showed high stability across a variety of temperatures, which might be advantageous for transportation and storage.

The clinical trials' main emphasis was on Neffy's effectiveness and comparability to injectable epinephrine, but researchers also closely examined the nasal spray formulation's potential side effects and safety issues. As with any drug, it's important for patients and healthcare professionals to be aware of any possible side effects.

Neffy's most often reported adverse effects in clinical studies were jitteriness, headache, tingling in the nose, throat irritation, and nasal pain. The majority of these adverse effects were minor and temporary, going away on their own. Crucially, they were mostly in line with the recognized adverse effects of adrenaline, independent of the mode of delivery. Neffy and injectable epinephrine's identical side effect profiles were considered a signpost for the safety profile of the nasal spray.

Because of the unique delivery method, researchers focused especially on local effects in the nasal cavity. Although a few subjects reported transient nose pain, there was no indication of significant or long-term harm to the nasal tissues. Long-term research will keep an eye out for any possible cumulative impacts on nasal health from regular usage.

One thing that became clear from the research was how pre-existing nasal issues may affect how effective Neffy is. Absorption rates varied between those who had nasal polyps or who had had nasal surgery. Based on these findings, it is advised that people with these illnesses speak with their doctors to see whether an injectable version of epinephrine might be a better fit for them.

The trials also looked at the possibility of systemic adverse effects, which are recognized consequences of adrenaline and included elevated blood pressure and heart rate. Since the frequency and intensity of these side effects were similar to those of injectable epinephrine, it seems that there were no additional systemic concerns associated with the nasal route of delivery.

The risk of an unintentional overdose was a crucial safety factor. It was discovered that this danger is reduced by the Neffy device's design, which administers a single, pre-measured dosage. As with any epinephrine product, however, the research stressed how crucial it is to have the right training and follow dosage recommendations.

The possibility of medication interactions was another issue that the study addressed. It is well recognized that epinephrine may interact with various drugs, especially beta-blockers and antidepressants. According to the research, there were no significant differences in these interactions between injectable and Neffy epinephrine, therefore medical professionals may use their current understanding of epinephrine interactions to the novel formulation.

Neffy took into account a few special factors, including how it may affect those who have asthma or respiratory allergies. Initially, there were doubts over the medication's appropriateness for those with nasal allergies since it is inhaled. Even in this demographic, the research revealed that Neffy was usually well-tolerated, however individual reactions may differ.

The possibility of tachyphylaxis, a condition in which taking a drug repeatedly eventually loses its effectiveness, was also investigated. This is a recognized risk factor for epinephrine, and research has not shown that administering the drug via the nose carries a higher risk of tachyphylaxis than does using an injectable version.

The safety studies' analysis of user mistake rates was one of their most intriguing features. Despite Neffy's ease of use, researchers wanted to know what may happen if it was administered incorrectly. Neffy provided therapeutic quantities of epinephrine in the majority of instances, even when it was used suboptimally—for example, by not inserting it all the way into the nose. The only difference could have been a slower rate of delivery. This resilience to real-world circumstances was considered a major benefit.

The environmental effect of Neffy in comparison to auto-injectors was also taken into account in the investigations. The single-use nasal spray device was shown to generate less plastic trash than standard auto-injectors, possibly providing an environmental advantage in light of the rising concerns around medical waste.

The psychological effects of administering an injection vs a nasal spray were also studied by researchers. When it came to utilizing Neffy, many participants felt less anxious than when they thought about giving themselves an injection. This decreased anxiety may result in quicker emergency care, which is essential for efficiently treating anaphylaxis.

The research also looked at how regular use of Neffy will affect people in the long run. Even though the acute safety profile was well established, longer-term follow-up studies were started by the researchers to keep an eye out for any possible cumulative effects, especially with regard to nose health and general epinephrine sensitivity.

One crucial finding from the research was the possibility of mishandling or abusing Neffy. There were worries that it would be used excessively or recreationally because of its non-invasive nature. In contrast to injectable epinephrine, the trials did not find any indication of an increased risk of abuse; nonetheless, continued surveillance and instruction were advised to guarantee appropriate usage.

The study also looked at Neffy's effectiveness in various age groups. Even though it was first approved for anyone above 66 pounds, research is still being done to see whether it may be used for newborns and younger children. These trials are essential to extending Neffy's potential user base and giving a needle-free choice to a larger spectrum of patients.

The potential use of Neffy in other medical circumstances, such as cardiac arrest, where quick epinephrine delivery is advantageous, is one area of continuing investigation. Neffy is a compelling candidate for investigation in these fields due to its simplicity of usage and quick absorption, even if these uses are currently purely speculative.

The investigations also looked at Neffy's affordability in comparison to conventional auto-injectors. In order to estimate the possible economic effect of broad Neffy use, researchers projected a number of scenarios, even though the ultimate cost was not decided during the clinical trials. In these economic assessments, variables including shorter training times, perhaps cheaper manufacturing costs, and the potential for higher medication adherence were all taken into account.

Neffy may help people in general become better prepared for anaphylaxis, according to some intriguing study findings. Researchers theorized that more individuals could be willing to get and carry epinephrine due to its simplicity of use and less anxiety associated with it. This might result in improved results in community settings where bystander intervention can be crucial.

The possibility of integrating Neffy into more comprehensive emergency response systems was also mentioned in the study. Research looked at the fastest way to teach first responders and school personnel to use Neffy, which might increase the number of people in the network who can save lives when severe allergic responses occur.

Chapter Four

Breaking Barriers in Anaphylaxis Treatment

Neffy, the first nasal spray authorized by the FDA to treat anaphylaxis, is a major advancement in emergency allergy therapy. This ground-breaking method offers a needle-free substitute for conventional epinephrine autoinjectors, addressing long-standing issues that have the potential to completely transform the way we treat severe allergic responses.

Trypanophobia, often known as needle phobia, is a dread that affects a significant section of the population. Estimates indicate that up to 10% of individuals may suffer from this phobia to some extent. This dread may have potentially fatal repercussions for those who suffer from severe allergies. Fear of needles may make using an autoinjector difficult and could dangerously delay giving epinephrine in anaphylactic situations. This problem is immediately addressed by Neffy's nasal spray format, which does away with the need for needle-based administration.

Beyond the acute anxiety of injection, needle phobia has psychological effects. Carrying and maybe utilizing an autoinjector is a source of worry and concern for many people with severe allergies. Constant concern may have a negative impact on quality of life by causing avoidance behaviors and decreased activity engagement. Neffy has the potential to lessen this psychological load by offering a needle-free solution, giving people greater self-assurance and readiness to control their allergies.

Children are especially going to gain a lot from this needle-free method. Managing allergies may be especially difficult for pediatric patients and their caretakers since these youngsters often show increased anxiety and resistance to injections. When a nasal spray is an option, younger people are more likely to follow emergency treatment procedures, which might save lives in dire circumstances.

Furthermore, the release of Neffy could persuade people who had previously refrained from getting prescriptions for epinephrine because they were afraid of needles to now get this life-saving drug. As a result, the allergic community may become more prepared, increasing the number of individuals with access to emergency care when necessary.

One cannot stress how convenient Neffy is to utilize in an emergency. Even though they work well, traditional autoinjectors need some experience and training to use properly. Even those who are used to using needles may find it difficult to give the injection correctly in high-stress emergency situations. Treatment mistakes or delays may be caused by a variety of factors, including garment obstacles, unintentional self-injection, or difficulties identifying the proper injection site.

Neffy's nasal spray format greatly streamlines the administration procedure. Most individuals find that utilizing a nasal spray is an intuitive behavior, which lowers the possibility of user mistake during crucial situations. This simplicity is especially helpful when unskilled onlookers are asked to help, or when the individual suffering anaphylaxis may need to self-administer the drug.

Another significant benefit of using Neffy is the possibility of quicker administration. Every second counts when treating anaphylaxis, so being able to provide the drug swiftly and effortlessly may have a big impact on how things turn out. When compared to an autoinjector, a nasal spray requires less preparation time, which might result in more rapid treatment and better patient results.

Moreover, the nasal spray format can lessen the reluctance that some people have when considering injecting themselves or others. Because of the lower psychological barrier, people may make decisions more quickly in emergency circumstances, taking the medicine as soon as they notice a strong allergic response instead of waiting to see whether their symptoms become worse.

Neffy's mobility and discretion add to its user-friendliness. Even though autoinjectors are meant to be portable, their size and shape may sometimes make them difficult to carry, particularly for those who want to travel light or don tight clothes. Because a nasal spray device is more recognizable and small, it may be easier to incorporate into everyday life, which increases the possibility that people will have the drug on hand when required.

Neffy has significantly more potential to improve public health than just its individual users. Neffy has the potential to enhance population-level anaphylaxis care by offering a less frightening and more approachable method of emergency allergy therapy.

Potentially more people at risk for anaphylaxis becoming epinephrine carriers is one of the biggest consequences for public health. According to current research, a large number of people who are given epinephrine autoinjectors may not carry them regularly or at all. While there are many other causes for this non-compliance, needle anxiety and discomfort are often mentioned as major ones. Through the removal of these obstacles, Neffy may increase the proportion of at-risk people who regularly carry their emergency medicine, which would lower the community's risk of untreated anaphylaxis.

The ease of use of Neffy's administration may potentially result in more epinephrine being accessible in public areas. Although a lot of restaurants, schools, and other public places have started carrying epinephrine autoinjectors, their broad usage may be hampered by the training needed to use them. Because nasal sprays are easier to apply, more places may decide to stock up on epinephrine and enable a larger group of people to help during crises.

Public education and understanding of anaphylaxis may be impacted by this improved accessibility and use. As more individuals become aware of the idea of using a nasal spray for allergic crises, discussions concerning severe allergic responses and how to manage them may be sparked. This increased awareness may help both those having reactions and bystanders identify anaphylactic symptoms more quickly and treat them more quickly.

It's also important to think about how Neffy may fit into larger emergency response plans. It may be simpler for emergency medical services, first responders, and even community people who have received first aid training to include a nasal spray in their emergency kits and protocols. Because of this, epinephrine may become more widely accessible in emergency circumstances, perhaps saving lives in instances where standard autoinjectors are unavailable or rescuers are reluctant to use them.

From the standpoint of public health policy, the release of Neffy could force recommendations and guidelines for the treatment of anaphylaxis to be reviewed. It could be necessary for medical authorities and associations to revise their guidelines to include nasal spray epinephrine in addition to autoinjectors as a primary therapeutic measure. This may result in population-level management of severe allergies that is more inclusive and thorough.

Neffy's financial effects on public health are noteworthy. The price of the drug is one consideration, but there is also a chance that more prompt and widespread use of epinephrine may result in fewer hospital stays and ER visits, which might save a significant amount of money on healthcare. Neffy may also lower the indirect expenses of lost work or school days owing to allergic responses if it improves the overall treatment of severe allergies.

Neffy's introduction has created research possibilities that may help us learn more about treating anaphylaxis. Research comparing the results of nasal spray delivery with conventional autoinjectors in practical situations may provide light on the relative efficacy of the various administration methods. Future treatment recommendations may benefit from this study, which may also spark new developments in the field of allergy care.

It's also important to think about how a needle-free epinephrine alternative would affect the world. A nasal spray substitute might greatly increase access to life-saving allergy therapy in areas where needle-based treatments are hindered by cultural or religious constraints. This could have a bigger effect in underdeveloped nations where it would be difficult to distribute and use autoinjectors logistically.

It will be essential to continuously check Neffy's performance in the actual world, just as with any new medical intervention. Important information on post-market surveillance's efficacy, safety profile, and potential pitfalls in usage will be available. This data will be essential for identifying any groups or circumstances in which conventional autoinjectors may still be preferred, as well as for continuously improving recommendations for its usage.

Important queries about patient education and training are also brought up by the introduction of Neffy. Even while the nasal spray format is often easier to use than an autoinjector, it is still important to make sure patients know how to administer the medication correctly. In order to teach patients how to utilize Neffy, healthcare practitioners will need to provide new teaching resources and methods. These may include simulation techniques or digital tools to improve learning.

Healthcare professionals will play a crucial role in helping patients decide between Neffy and conventional autoinjectors. The best choice for each individual will depend on a number of factors, including lifestyle considerations, unique allergy profiles, and patient preferences. This individualized strategy to manage anaphylaxis may improve overall results and patient satisfaction.

Beyond only the short-term health advantages, Neffy may also help those with severe allergies live better lives. Having a needle-free alternative might provide psychological comfort and lessen the stress and anxiety related to managing allergies, which could enhance the population's mental health results. Although less obvious than its physiological benefits, this part of Neffy's influence may be just as important for allergy patients' long-term health.

It will be fascinating to see how Neffy integrates into many facets of society as it gets more accessible. To include this new option, schools may need to revise their staff training protocols and allergy action plans. Neffy will also need to be taken into account when making plans for public spaces such as restaurants, airplanes, and other establishments that follow procedures for managing allergic reactions.

Neffy's creation and certification also establish a standard for innovation in the distribution of emergency medications. This discovery may spur more investigation into other ways to administer other emergency drugs, which might result in a new generation of accessible, needle-free treatments for a range of ailments.

Neffy's ability to surmount obstacles to anaphylactic therapy may potentially have wider ramifications for how we build medication delivery systems and medical devices. This nasal spray format's focus on accessibility and user experience may have an impact on future advancements in a variety of healthcare domains, encouraging a more patient-centered approach to medical technology.

The long-term effects of Neffy on anaphylaxis outcomes will be a major subject of investigation going forward. Neffy's usefulness in the real world will be better understood by longitudinal studies comparing the frequency and severity of anaphylactic responses in people having access to it with those using conventional autoinjectors. These investigations can possibly highlight unforeseen advantages or difficulties related to the widespread use of epinephrine nasal spray.

Neffy has the power to alter how the general public views severe allergies and how they should be treated. The shame and anxiety attached to carrying and utilizing emergency allergy medicine may fade as needle-free choices proliferate. This might result in a more inclusive atmosphere in public areas, businesses, and schools as well as more social acceptance and support for those dealing with severe allergies.

Chapter Five

Practical Aspects of Neffy

Neffy is a needle-free substitute for conventional epinephrine autoinjectors, marking a substantial progress in the management of severe allergic responses. The nasal spray formulation possibly improves access to life-saving therapy during anaphylactic situations by addressing several practical difficulties that patients and caregivers experience with injectable epinephrine.

User-friendliness has been taken into consideration while designing the dose and administration of Neffy. One nasal spray dosage of epinephrine is included in each Neffy device. Neffy is now authorized by the FDA for usage in adults and children above the weight of thirty kilos (66 pounds). One spray into one nostril is the suggested dosage for these people. Users no longer have to deal with needles or monitor dosages thanks to this simple administration technique, which may be especially helpful in high-stress emergency scenarios.

The simplicity of usage of Neffy's nasal spray style is one of its main benefits. Neffy's manufacturer, ARS Pharmaceuticals, found that in tests, untrained people could accurately administer the medication in emergency situations without any previous training. This simplicity of use may be essential in cases when the individual suffering from anaphylaxis is unable to give themselves the medicine and someone else has to assist.

It's crucial to remember that, similar to injectable epinephrine, Neffy may sometimes need a second dosage. Regardless of whether they have taken Neffy or an injectable type of epinephrine, the FDA advises individuals suffering anaphylaxis to seek emergency medical attention for careful monitoring. By taking this precaution, people may be guaranteed complete care and be watched for any possible symptom recurrence or need for further treatment.

Neffy isn't for everyone, even if it has a lot of benefits. The FDA has warned that those who have had nasal surgery or who have certain nasal problems, such polyps, may not be able to absorb Neffy well enough. To find out whether injectable epinephrine is a better alternative for them, these people should speak with their medical professionals. This emphasizes how crucial customized medical guidance is for treating severe allergies and selecting the best emergency care alternatives.

Neffy's storage and shelf life are noticeably better than those of conventional epinephrine autoinjectors.

Compared to many autoinjectors, which typically have a shelf life of 18 months, Neffy has a 30-month shelf life. For patients and healthcare systems, this longer shelf life may result in savings on waste and fewer prescription renewals, which would be convenient and cost-effective.

Regardless of the form, epinephrine must be stored properly to retain its effectiveness. Neffy's particular storage instructions were not included in the material that was supplied, but it is probable that they will be comparable to those for other products that contain epinephrine. Generally speaking, epinephrine has to be kept out of direct sunlight, at normal temperature, and shielded from very cold or very hot conditions. Neffy's extended shelf life might perhaps reduce the anxiety that comes with constantly monitoring expiry dates and swapping out outdated gadgets.

Neffy's possible influence on anaphylaxis therapy depends in large part on its availability and cost. Neffy is anticipated to be accessible in the US eight weeks after receiving FDA clearance, according to ARS Pharmaceuticals. This timescale is comparatively short, indicating that the corporation has made preparations for manufacturing and distribution in advance of approval, which may assist satisfy early demand.

At the time of the FDA announcement, ARS Pharmaceuticals had not released Neffy's list price. Richard Lowenthal, the CEO of the firm, did, however, remark that the cost to insurance would be comparable to that of Auvi-Q, another epinephrine auto injector, which was reported to cost around $640. Neffy is expected to be positioned as a premium product in the epinephrine market, according to this price strategy.

A number of measures have been suggested by ARS Pharmaceuticals to address cost and access problems. The business intends to provide a co-pay scheme that would cap out-of-pocket expenses for two single-use devices at $25 for those with commercial insurance that supports Neffy. Many patients' financial burdens might be greatly lessened by this initiative, increasing Neffy's accessibility for those with insurance coverage.

A price option of $199 for two doses of Neffy has been released by ARS Pharmaceuticals for people without insurance or those with significant out-of-pocket expenses. Even while this is still a high price, it is far less than the full list price, which may help some patients who would not otherwise be able to afford epinephrine autoinjectors get the drug.

Additionally, ARS Pharmaceuticals has committed to giving Neffy out for free to those people who are unable to pay for the medication. For individuals who are most in need, our patient assistance program may be essential in ensuring that access to this potentially life-saving drug is not impeded by financial difficulties.

Neffy's price and access policies are in line with a larger pharmaceutical industry trend that seeks to strike a balance between patient access and profitability. The goal of the tiered pricing strategy is to keep the prescription affordable for a broad patient base while yet retaining its market value. It includes insurance coverage, cash pay choices, and patient aid programs.

The market study conducted by ARS Pharmaceuticals indicates that there is a sizable potential market for Neffy. According to the business, 3.2 million people—including kids who are afraid of needles—strongly detest autoinjectors and may swiftly convert to the nasal spray style. Neffy may also be preferred by an additional 3.3 million individuals who have prescriptions for injectable epinephrine written but haven't filled them.

Most importantly, according to ARS Pharmaceuticals, 13.5 million individuals have been diagnosed with anaphylaxis but have never been given an epinephrine prescription. The provision of a simpler, needle-free substitute would motivate these people to acquire and carry emergency epinephrine, which might improve the prognosis in situations involving severe allergic responses.

The company's high expectations for Neffy's acceptance are reminiscent of the widespread use of nasal-spray naloxone, or Narcan, to reverse opiate overdoses. About 80% of naloxone uses are made via Narcan, and ARS Pharmaceuticals predicts that Neffy will be adopted at a rate comparable to that of the epinephrine market. Based on this comparison, a lot of people and healthcare professionals may end up choosing the nasal spray format.

Neffy may be used for purposes other than individual prescriptions. Neffy may eventually be included in airline emergency kits, according to ARS Pharmaceuticals' conversations with manufacturers of such kits. Neffy may also be available in public spaces like restaurants, just as automatic external defibrillators (AEDs) are in many public locations these days.

Neffy's simplicity of use is supported by its potential for broader public access, as shown by the company's research with persons who are not trained. The capacity of bystanders to accurately administer the drug without any previous training may play a major role in improving outcomes in public places where emergency medical assistance may not be readily accessible.

Future plans for ARS Pharmaceuticals include extending Neffy's authorized use to younger kids. By the end of the third quarter of 2024, the business plans to apply for FDA clearance for use in youngsters weighing between 33 and 66 pounds (15 to 30 kilograms). The potential user base for Neffy would be significantly increased by this lower-dose variant, which would be comparable to the junior versions of the present epinephrine autoinjectors.

Neffy's entry into the anaphylactic treatment industry is probably going to have repercussions for the whole healthcare system. Neffy will need familiarity with emergency rooms, allergists, and primary care physicians in order to prescribe and instruct patients on its usage. Neffy training is also required for school nurses and other caregivers who are often in charge of giving children's emergency drugs.

Neffy's clearance could encourage further advancements in the realm of treating allergies and anaphylaxis. Rival pharmaceutical firms could be inspired to create their own needle-free substitutes or enhance the designs of already-available autoinjectors. Through more alternatives and better technology, patients may benefit from this competition's potential to significantly develop epinephrine delivery systems.

Neffy's effectiveness could promote studies into additional emergency drug delivery methods that do not need needles. If the nasal spray format for epinephrine administration works well and becomes widely used, it may pave the way for similar methods to be used in the treatment of other acute illnesses that are presently treated with injectable drugs.

Data from real-world use cases and Neffy's success will be critical as the tool becomes more widely accessible. Neffy's performance outside of clinical trial settings, particularly its adaptability to different climatic circumstances and its influence on patient outcomes in real anaphylaxis instances, will be extensively documented by post-market monitoring and investigations.

Neffy's launch marks a substantial advancement in the management of anaphylaxis by providing a needle-free alternative that may increase accessibility to life-saving drugs and lessen reluctance to administer epinephrine in an emergency. Its practical features—such as its longer shelf life, ease of administration, and attempts to maintain affordability—place it in a position to possibly revolutionize allergy emergency treatment.

Chapter Six

Special Populations and Considerations

Special populations in the field of anaphylactic therapy need to be carefully considered. Specialized strategies are necessary to address the particular issues faced by children and persons with nasal disorders. Neffy, an innovative nasal spray epinephrine, presents these organizations with new opportunities as well as significant concerns.

Usage in Children

Neffy offers a potentially revolutionary approach to managing pediatric anaphylaxis, since children are more susceptible to severe allergic responses. Neffy's FDA clearance for children over 66 pounds is a big step forward, but it's important to know the subtleties of using it with smaller populations.

The dread of needles in youngsters may be a significant obstacle to giving them adrenaline on time. This issue is immediately addressed by Neffy's nasal spray style, which may make it more likely that kids or their caretakers would take the drug as soon as it's required. In an emergency, when every second matters, this might save lives.

Nevertheless, younger or smaller children are left out of the existing approval, which is only for youngsters above 66 pounds. Neffy's manufacturer, ARS Pharmaceuticals, intends to apply for FDA clearance for use in kids weighing 33 to 66 pounds. This needle-free option's potential reach might be greatly increased, but it also raises concerns regarding dosage and administration for tiny bodies.

Children's nasal spray epinephrine pharmacokinetics may vary from adults', therefore careful research and maybe modified dose regimens are required. Children's nasal channel size, mucus production, and general absorption rates are among the factors that need to be taken into account. Clear standards for pediatric usage must be established as research advances to guarantee that children get the right dosage of medicine for anaphylactic therapy.

Also, Neffy's child-friendly interface has to be taken into consideration. Although administering medication using a nasal spray may seem less daunting than using an auto-injector, correct technique is still essential. It will be crucial that children and the people who look for them get education and training. This entails educating parents, teachers, and other caregivers on proper administration of the spray in addition to teaching kids how to administer it on their own when they're old enough.

Another crucial factor to take into account is how Neffy can affect the policies and practices of schools regarding the treatment of anaphylaxis. There are procedures in place in many schools for handling and storing epinephrine auto-injectors. These policies may need to be updated in light of the availability of nasal sprays. This may include making changes to emergency response plans and providing training for school personnel.

It will be vital to do long-term research on children's nasal epinephrine usage. Even while preliminary evidence indicates that injectable epinephrine is equally effective, further study should concentrate on any possible variations in results, adverse effects, or long-term consequences that are unique to pediatric groups. Ensuring the highest standards of safety and effectiveness and improving recommendations for use in children will be made possible with the use of this data.

One should not undervalue the psychological effects of giving children an auto-injector as opposed to a nasal spray. Having an epinephrine auto-injector on hand might cause anxiety or make many kids with severe allergies feel different from their classmates. Some of these worries could be allayed by a nasal spray alternative, which might enhance quality of life and adherence to carrying emergency medicine.

Pediatric allergists and immunologists will be key players in deciding where Neffy fits into children's severe allergy treatment plans when the device becomes more generally accessible. When choosing between Neffy and conventional auto-injectors, they will need to take the child's age, size, ability to follow directions, and any coinciding medical issues into account.

More research should be done on the possibility of using Neffy with extremely young children, especially those who are under the current weight barrier. In babies and toddlers, for whom giving an injection may be very difficult, it might completely transform the treatment of anaphylaxis if further study confirms its safety and effectiveness in this age range.

Nasal Disorders and Notifications

While many people find Neffy to be a suitable substitute, there are special concerns for those who have specific nasal disorders. Many nasal problems may affect the appropriate absorption of epinephrine via the nasal mucosa, which is crucial to the efficiency of a nasal spray.

Nose congestion is one of the main issues. Nasal passages may swell and congest during an allergic response, which might interfere with the absorption of epinephrine injected by the nose. This calls into doubt Neffy's dependability in these kinds of circumstances. Individuals who have persistent nose congestion, stemming from allergies, anatomical problems, or other circumstances, need to thoroughly assess whether a nasal spray is the most suitable choice for meeting their immediate epidural requirements.

Nasal polyps are an additional problem. These benign tumors in the nasal airways may block airflow and perhaps affect how well drugs injected via the nose are distributed and absorbed. Whether a person has nasal polyps, they should speak with their doctor to see whether Neffy is a good fit or if injectable epinephrine is a better alternative.

A previous history of nose surgery is an additional issue that has to be carefully considered. Modifications to the nasal structure resulting from medical or cosmetic treatments may affect how well a nasal spray drug works. Individuals who have had nasal surgery should talk to their ENT or allergist about the consequences to make sure that Neffy is a good fit for their anaphylactic treatment strategy.

Neffy usage may also be impacted by chronic sinusitis, a disorder marked by inflammation of the sinus cavities. Patients with chronic sinusitis may have different nasal environments, which might affect how well nasally given epinephrine is absorbed and distributed. To ascertain if a nasal spray formulation would be as beneficial in these individuals' cases as an injectable one, further assessment may be required.

A frequent issue called deviated septum, in which the nasal septum is notably off-center, may affect how evenly a nasal spray drug is distributed. Given their unique nasal structure, patients with this illness may need to examine whether Neffy can be delivered and absorbed consistently.

It is important to use caution while using a nasal spray medicine for those who have epistaxis, or repeated nosebleeds. The strong spray may worsen the propensity to bleed from the nose, and blood in the nasal passages may interfere with the absorption of medicines. Together with their medical professionals, these patients should carefully consider the advantages and disadvantages of utilizing Neffy vs injectable epinephrine.

Although anosmia, or the lack of smell, does not directly decrease Neffy's efficacy, it may interfere with a patient's ability to determine if the drug has been given correctly. This may be especially important in high-stress emergency scenarios when effective management is essential.

Another crucial factor to think about is the use of additional nasal drugs. For the treatment of allergies, many people utilize antihistamine sprays or nasal corticosteroids. It is important to thoroughly research and comprehend the interactions between these drugs and Neffy, especially with regard to their efficacy and absorption.

Extreme dryness or high humidity are two examples of environmental conditions that may impact nasal passageways and determine how effective a nasal spray epinephrine is. Patients may need to think about how their anaphylaxis treatment strategy may be affected by living in or visiting places with notable climatic changes.

It is important to carefully consider if a nasal spray epinephrine option is acceptable for those who have a history of cocaine use or misuse, since this drug may cause serious harm to nasal tissues. In these situations, the nasal environment changes may have an impact on how well Neffy is absorbed and works.

Nasal spray drugs may provide particular difficulties for patients with autoimmune diseases that damage the nasal mucosa, such as Wegener's granulomatosis (previously known as granulomatosis with polyangiitis). Neffy's efficacy in each of these circumstances should be carefully evaluated on an individual basis.

It is necessary to continue researching the possibility of local irritation or unfavorable responses in the nasal passages while using Neffy often. The drug is meant to be used in an emergency, but those who have had many severe allergic responses may need to take it more often, and the long-term consequences on nasal tissues should be watched closely.

The effectiveness of a nasal spray in treating severe responses involving the upper airway, such as angioedema of the mouth and throat, should be carefully considered for individuals having a history of these reactions. Neffy's blood levels of epinephrine are equivalent to those of injectable formulations, however in situations where there is extensive upper airway involvement, the mode of administration may play a crucial role in the treatment plan.

Neffy usage has to be evaluated specifically in individuals with additional nasal problems, such as pyriform aperture stenosis or choanal atresia. The administration and efficacy of a nasal spray drug may be impacted by certain uncommon disorders that alter nasal architecture.

The possibility of allergic responses to Neffy's constituent parts has to be taken into account, just like with any drug. Although it is uncommon, those who have a history of allergic reactions to any of the chemicals in the nasal spray formulation should refrain from using it and instead utilize other ways to administer epinephrine.

Another thing to think about is how altitude affects the efficacy of nasal spray medications. Patients who reside in mountainous regions or often travel to high-altitude settings may need to talk with their healthcare professionals about whether taking Neffy in these situations calls for any changes to their anaphylactic treatment strategy.

When nasal cauterization is performed on a patient for nosebleeds or other causes, the nasal tissue environment is changed, which may impact the way nasal drugs are absorbed. To confirm Neffy's efficacy in their particular situation, some individuals would need to undergo further testing.

Another area that needs careful examination is the use of Neffy in patients with vasomotor rhinitis, a disorder marked by runny nose and nasal congestion from oversensitive blood vessels in the nose. These individuals' modified nasal environments may have an influence on how well a nasal spray containing epinephrine is absorbed and works.

The distribution and absorption of a nasal spray drug may be affected in individuals having a history of nasal trauma or fractures due to modifications in their nasal architecture. Neffy may not be the best choice for these people; a complete examination of the nasal passages may be required.

An essential practical concern is how frequent upper respiratory infections can affect Neffy's efficacy. When a patient has nasal congestion from a cold or the flu, they need clear instructions on whether to use Neffy or switch to an injectable alternative.

Neffy usage may need to be done with caution in people who have chronic rhinosinusitis with nasal polyps (CRSwNP), a disorder that may drastically change nasal structure and function. Careful assessment is necessary to determine the nasal spray's efficacy when widespread polyp illness is present.

An intriguing topic for research is the use of Neffy in patients receiving immunotherapy for nasal allergies. Analyzing the potential interactions between nasally delivered epinephrine and the altered immune response in the nasal passages may help improve the treatment of anaphylaxis in these individuals.

Chapter Seven

The Future of Anaphylaxis Management

With Neffy's clearance, a major advancement in the treatment of anaphylaxis has been made, creating new opportunities for emergency allergy care. With more treatment options becoming available and perhaps broader uses in the works, the field of managing anaphylaxis is set to undergo significant change in the near future.

Policymakers, pharmaceutical corporations, and healthcare practitioners all agree that increasing access to anaphylactic therapy is an important objective. Fear of injections is one of the main obstacles to timely treatment that is addressed by the development of a needle-free alternative. The fear that is especially common in children and some adults has caused delays in the delivery of life-saving epinephrine in the past. Neffy might significantly lessen this challenge.

Because nasal spray administration is so simple to use, people who are given emergency epinephrine may utilize it more often. Millions of people with anaphylaxis diagnosis, according to ARS Pharmaceuticals, the company that makes Neffy, have never had a prescription for emergency epinephrine written. Healthcare professionals may be more inclined to prescribe it if a nasal spray alternative is available because they may assume that patients would carry and use it more often.

Furthermore, the possibility of distributing Neffy more widely in public areas might greatly improve readiness for emergencies. Neffy may end up in the same places where automated external defibrillators (AEDs) are already often found—schools, airports, and other public places. Neffy may be seen at restaurants, retail stores, and entertainment venues in addition to first aid kits, offering an extra degree of protection for those with severe allergies.

The aviation sector has already shown interest in integrating Neffy into aircraft emergency medical kits. For passengers with severe allergies, this might be a game-changer, providing peace of mind and perhaps preventing crises mid-flight. Neffy's needle-free shape and small size make it especially ideal for these kinds of small areas.

In order to increase access to this new therapeutic option, education will be vital. Campaigns to educate the public about the symptoms of anaphylaxis and the availability of nasal spray treatments might enable bystanders to intervene in life-threatening circumstances. Like the popular use of naloxone nasal spray for opioid overdose reversal, the intuitive nature of nasal spray administration may facilitate aid from untrained persons.

In-depth Neffy training will be necessary for medical staff in order to guarantee that patients are properly educated. This entails being aware of the ideal method of administration, the needs for storage, and any possible drawbacks with the nasal spray type. To optimize the advantages of this cutting-edge therapy, further professional education will be crucial, just as with any new medical intervention.

Neffy's acceptance for adults and kids weighing more than 66 pounds is only the start. By pursuing clearance for usage in younger children, ARS Pharmaceuticals hopes to further transform the treatment of pediatric anaphylaxis. For young children, the idea of a needle-free solution is especially appealing since it might reduce a lot of the worry that comes with carrying and utilizing emergency epinephrine in this susceptible group.

Neffy's advancement not only increases accessibility but also creates opportunities for broader uses in allergy therapy. Research into other drugs that could benefit from this mode of administration may be sparked by the effectiveness of a nasal spray formulation for the delivery of epinephrine. For example, nasal spray formulations of antihistamines or corticosteroids, which are used in allergy therapy, may be a good option since they might function more quickly or provide patients with more convenience.

Neffy's invention may potentially open the door to improvements in other emergency medical fields. Should the nasal spray demonstrate its efficacy and dependability in administering epinephrine, scientists may investigate analogous methodologies for other urgent pharmaceuticals. This may result in a new wave of simple, quick-acting medications for a range of acute ailments.

Neffy's success might spur immunotherapy researchers to develop nasal spray formulations for allergy desensitization therapies. While the majority of immunotherapy treatments available today require injections or sublingual tablets, a nasal spray would provide a more practical and perhaps more efficient way to administer allergens for the aim of desensitization.

Neffy's capacity for self-administration fits well with larger healthcare trends that support patient autonomy and chronic disease self-management. When patients get more used to the concept of self-administering emergency drugs, more self-administered remedies for other ailments may be developed, which in certain circumstances may eliminate the need for emergency medical attention.

Future research and improvement in the treatment of anaphylaxis will greatly benefit from the data gathered from the actual usage of Neffy in the field. Researchers will learn more about the nasal spray's efficiency, usability, and potential drawbacks when more patients use it in real emergency scenarios. Future developments in the composition and administration of epinephrine may result from the guidance provided by this data, which might lead to ever more sophisticated therapies.

Neffy's success may potentially increase competition in the pharmaceutical sector by motivating other businesses to spend money on developing substitute epinephrine delivery systems. This rivalry may spur innovation and result in a wide range of anaphylaxis treatment choices, each tailored to the unique requirements and preferences of the patient.

Regarding public health, the launch of Neffy may have significant consequences. The nasal spray format may lower the overall incidence of severe anaphylactic outcomes if it does encourage more people to carry and utilize emergency epinephrine. As more patients are handled well in the community, this might lessen the demand on emergency medical services and hospital emergency rooms.

Another crucial factor to take into account is the possibility of cost reductions in the healthcare system. Neffy's adoption will be influenced by its initial cost, but there may be a big long-term economic benefit. Neffy has the potential to save healthcare systems and insurance companies a significant amount of money if it lowers the need for acute medical treatments for anaphylaxis and avoids hospitalizations.

It will be essential to keep a careful eye on Nelly's real-world performance as it becomes more accessible. Important information on its safety profile, efficacy, and any uncommon side events that may not have been seen in clinical studies will be obtained via post-market surveillance. Its further assessment will be crucial to improving use instructions and guaranteeing its seamless incorporation into anaphylactic treatment procedures.

It's also important to think about how Neffy's acceptance in the US may affect other countries. Other nations may accelerate their own approval procedures for comparable medications as they see the introduction and uptake of this new therapeutic option. This may cause a change in the way anaphylaxis is managed globally, making needle-free choices the standard rather than the exception.

Personalized medicine techniques may potentially lead to breakthroughs in the treatment of anaphylaxis in the future. With increasing knowledge of the genetic and environmental variables that lead to severe allergic responses, Neffy-like therapies may be customized to the specific needs of each patient. This might include modifying doses or creating formulations that are tailored to certain patient subgroups according to their distinct qualities.

Another promising development for the treatment of anaphylaxis in the future is the incorporation of technology. It is not unimaginable for smart gadgets to recognize the early warning indicators of an allergic response, notify emergency contacts automatically, or even deliver epinephrine on their own. Neffy's creation may serve as a prototype for these kinds of sophisticated, all-in-one allergy control solutions.

The FDA's clearance of Neffy after its successful clinical trials might hasten the investigation of other epinephrine delivery methods. Although the nasal spray is a big step forward, researchers may look at other non-invasive delivery techniques like inhalation devices or transdermal patches to provide patients and medical professionals even more choices.

Future research on anaphylaxis remedies may potentially take the environment into account. Manufacturers may concentrate on creating environmentally friendly packaging and delivery technologies for emergency pharmaceuticals like Neffy as sustainability plays a bigger role in healthcare. This might lessen the negative effects of these life-saving medicines on the environment by using recyclable or biodegradable components.

Another topic that is worth investigating is the possibility of integrating telemedicine with novel therapies for anaphylaxis. Patients using Neffy-like devices may be able to get real-time advice from medical experts in the event of an allergic reaction as remote healthcare services advance. To guarantee correct administration and follow-up treatment, this may include video consultations or AI-powered support.

Education systems may develop to include instruction on novel anaphylactic therapies, such as Neffy.

Comprehensive allergy management programs that involve practical instruction using nasal spray epinephrine devices might be implemented in workplaces, schools, and community groups. This extensive education program may raise awareness of allergies and equip people to handle anaphylactic shock situations.

Neffy's advancement may have an impact on food industry procedures as well. It is possible that food producers and restaurants would feel more comfortable broadening their offers to include items that have historically been avoided owing to allergy concerns if there is a readily available and perhaps more accessible emergency treatment alternative. This would, however, need to be carefully balanced with a persistent focus on allergy knowledge and avoidance.

With the release of Neffy, research into the long-term implications of frequent epinephrine usage could pick up steam. Because of its alleged reduced barrier to use, the nasal spray format may lead to more frequent administration of epinephrine in non-emergency scenarios. Therefore, it will become more crucial to comprehend the effects of increased epinephrine exposure.

In order to offer thorough care of severe allergic responses, combination therapies that combine longer-acting medications with fast-acting epinephrine, such as Neffy, may potentially be developed in the future. This may include using nasal sprays to relieve symptoms right away as well as taking drugs to lessen inflammation or stop symptoms from coming back.

New understandings of the processes behind anaphylaxis might result in innovative therapeutic modalities that, in some situations, could replace or supplement epinephrine as immunology progresses. Long-term anaphylaxis care may change as a result of research into tailored medicines that target the underlying causes of severe allergic responses, even if epinephrine will probably continue to be the go-to medication for emergency treatment in the near future.

Increased financing and research into allergy prevention may result from Neffy's success in addressing one facet of allergy management: emergency therapy. This may result in developments in early intervention techniques, enhanced diagnostic instruments, and maybe even approaches to stop or reverse the onset of severe allergies.

In summary, the treatment of anaphylaxis has a promising future. Neffy's arrival not only offers a fresh course of therapy but also raises the possibility of a paradigm change in the way we handle urgent allergy care. We may look forward to a day when managing severe allergic responses will be easier, with fewer obstacles to treatment and better patient outcomes, as access increases and new uses are developed. In the years to come, it's possible that the path that started with the approval of the first nasal spray epinephrine may lead to even more ground-breaking and life-saving discoveries.

Conclusion

A New Era in Allergy Emergency Care

We're clearly seeing a big change in allergy emergency treatment when we consider the ground-breaking launch of Neffy, the first FDA-approved nasal spray epinephrine for severe allergic responses. With this revolutionary discovery, a new era that promises to revolutionize the way we treat and manage anaphylaxis has begun.

Neffy has the potential to have a significant and wide-ranging influence on the field of allergy therapy. For many years, injectable epinephrine—most often in the form of auto-injectors like EpiPen—has been the standard of treatment for treating anaphylaxis. Undoubtedly, these gadgets have saved numerous lives, but they have also made it more difficult for people to receive treatment on time, especially for those who are afraid of needles or are reluctant to utilize injectable devices.

An alternate nasal spray has been introduced to directly address these problems. Neffy eliminates a major psychological barrier—the need for a needle—that has often resulted in risky delays in giving out life-saving medicine. Faster treatment times at crucial periods when every second matters might arise from this. A nasal spray's simplicity of application may also make it more likely for onlookers to intervene in an emergency and save lives, especially in public places where qualified medical personnel may not be instantly accessible.

Furthermore, Neffy's endorsement makes epinephrine more widely available. More at-risk people may choose to regularly carry the medicine with them because of its user-friendly design. Since more individuals will have instant access to the necessary therapy, this enhanced readiness might considerably lower the probability of deadly anaphylactic responses.

The possible effects might affect not only specific individuals but also the larger healthcare system. If more patients can successfully self-administer medication at the first indication of a response, emergency rooms could notice a decrease in severe instances of anaphylaxis. This may result in lower medical expenses and less demand on emergency services.

Neffy might provide school nurses and staff a less scary way to manage allergic responses in educational settings, where food allergies are becoming a rising problem. This might improve outcomes for allergic adolescents by enabling schools to respond to anaphylaxis with more assurance and speed.

Neffy's clearance establishes a precedent for the pharmaceutical industry by proving that other means of delivering emergency drugs may be both viable and acceptable. This discovery might spur additional advancements in drug delivery technologies in a range of therapeutic domains, which could result in more patient-friendly alternatives for other essential drugs.

Neffy's launch is probably only the start of a long line of advancements in allergy therapy, as we look to the future. The effectiveness of this nasal spray epinephrine may open up new avenues for investigation into non-injectable emergency drugs, not just for allergies but also for other acute illnesses.

A region that might be developed is the extension of Neffy's permitted applications. Although it is presently only licensed for adults and children over 66 pounds, further study might result in formulations that are appropriate for newborns and smaller children. This would fill a significant need in the available therapeutic choices, as giving injections to very young infants may be very difficult.

Creating formulations that last longer might be another opportunity for innovation. Neffy is an epinephrine auto-injector with a 30-month shelf life, compared to the average of around 18 months for current models. This might be extended much longer in the future, therefore minimizing the frequency of replacement and perhaps the patients' long-term expenditures.

Neffy's success could encourage studies into other ways to provide comparable emergency drugs, such as epinephrine. There may be upcoming sublingual pills, transdermal patches, or even inhalable formulations, each with its own advantages regarding user-friendliness, rate of action, or compatibility for certain patient demographics.

The area of allergy therapy is ripe for innovation, even outside the realm of epinephrine. Neffy's success was built on three key features: simplicity of use, less patient anxiety, and quick response. These features might be extended to other areas of allergy care. For example, more accessible immunotherapy alternatives may emerge, going beyond standard allergy needles to include sublingual pills or other non-invasive techniques.

Technological developments are also anticipated to have a big impact on allergy therapy in the future. In order to provide real-time advice during an allergic response, smart auto-injectors or nasal spray devices may include features like dosage monitoring, automated emergency alerts, or smartphone connectivity. These technologically advanced gadgets have the potential to enhance the efficacy of therapy as well as data collection on the occurrence and consequences of anaphylaxis.

Treatment for allergies may potentially benefit from the customized medicine sector. More specialized treatments may be developed as our knowledge of the genetic and environmental components that cause allergies increases. This may result in the development of personalized allergy profiles for each patient, which might lead to improved allergic response management and prevention.

The field of early diagnosis and prevention presents another opportunity for innovation. Managing allergies might be revolutionized by wearable technology or biosensors that identify early indications of an allergic response before they worsen. By warning the user to take precautions or start treatment as soon as feasible, these gadgets may be able to stop full-blown anaphylaxis.

The popularity of Neffy could hasten the investigation of the fundamental causes of acute allergic responses. The physiology of anaphylaxis and the ways in which various delivery techniques impact the body's reaction may be better understood by scientists when more information on the efficacy of nasal epinephrine delivery becomes accessible. This may eventually result in even more potent medicines.

Neffy's debut may lead to new public health campaigns focused on raising allergy awareness and enhancing emergency readiness. Employees in restaurants, schools, and other establishments that interact with the public may get further training on how to identify and handle severe allergic reactions. Since giving a nasal spray is easier than giving an injection, this kind of training may be more popular and successful.

Neffy's achievement is likely to be noticed by the pharmaceutical industry, which might result in more funding for allergy research and development. This may lead to a more varied pipeline of allergy medicines, providing a greater selection of alternatives for patients and healthcare professionals to choose from according to their unique requirements and preferences.

With allergy rates rising everywhere, especially in industrialized nations, there will probably be a greater need for novel therapies. In order to combat the expanding allergy pandemic, this may encourage further cooperation between pharmaceutical corporations, scholarly researchers, and public health groups. These collaborations might result in innovations in early intervention and preventive techniques in addition to therapy.

With the introduction of products like Neffy, the regulatory environment governing allergy medications may potentially change. It is possible that regulatory bodies may create new policies and procedures for approving unconventional means of administering emergency drugs. This may simplify the procedure for releasing comparable inventions into the market in the future.

The effectiveness of patient-friendly therapies like Neffy may have an impact on how other chronic illnesses are managed in the larger healthcare system. A broad variety of therapeutic domains might benefit from the use of design concepts that lower adherence barriers and enable patients to take charge of their own health management.

Going ahead, we should think about how breakthroughs like Neffy will affect the world. Even though they were first licensed in the US, everyone needs better allergy remedies. In countries with limited healthcare resources, the development of affordable, portable, and user-friendly methods for delivering epinephrine might have a major impact and perhaps save lives in places where standard auto-injectors may be hard to come by or prohibitively costly.

The key to optimizing the advantages of these breakthroughs will be raising awareness and promoting education. Patients, caregivers, and healthcare professionals will need extensive education programs as new treatment alternatives become accessible. In addition to teaching students how to use new devices properly, these programs must stress the need of receiving treatment as soon as possible and how to recognize the signs of anaphylaxis.

Innovations such as Neffy have a significant psychological influence that should not be overlooked. The worry of an allergic response and the burden of carrying and maybe utilizing an auto-injector can significantly lower quality of life for a large number of people with severe allergies. More approachable therapy alternatives could lessen this psychological load and help allergy sufferers live more confidently and worry-free.

It will be critical to keep an eye on these new technologies' long-term impacts and safety profiles as we use them. Maintaining the highest standards of safety and effectiveness for novel therapies like Neffy will need continuous research and post-market supervision.

Improvements in other areas of medical science are also expected to have an impact on the field of allergy research. For example, advances in immunology may provide fresh perspectives on the processes behind allergic responses, perhaps creating whole new therapeutic and preventive opportunities. Similar to this, advancements in areas like medication delivery systems and nanotechnology may be used to produce allergy therapies that are even more precise and potent.

It's obvious that Neffy's clearance signifies more than simply a new therapeutic option as we look to the future. It represents a change in the way we think about medical breakthroughs, putting the needs of the patient and practicality ahead of clinical effectiveness. Future advancements in a variety of medical specialties are probably going to be influenced by this patient-centric approach to medication development and distribution.

The path that resulted in Neffy's clearance also emphasizes how crucial perseverance and originality are to medical research. Researchers faced considerable obstacles in creating an epinephrine nasal spray formulation that could equal the effectiveness of injectable forms, but they were motivated to discover answers by the possible advantages. We will need to maintain this innovative and tenacious mindset as we work to address the many obstacles that allergies and other medical issues provide.

As we approach this new chapter in allergy emergency care, it's critical to understand that while breakthroughs like Neffy signify a great deal of advancement, they cannot treat allergies. The ultimate objective is still to discover strategies to stop allergies from ever occurring in the first place or to treat them once they have. In this context, it will be vital to continue studying the immunological tolerance mechanisms and the underlying causes of allergies.

In summary, the approval of Neffy heralds the start of an exciting new era in allergy medicine. Its potential significance goes much beyond only offering an improvement over epinephrine auto-injectors. It signifies a paradigm change in the way we handle emergency drugs by placing a strong emphasis on patient empowerment and usability. With an eye toward the future, we may expect a surge of developments motivated by the ideas of efficacy, accessibility, and patient-centric design that will continue to enhance the lives of people with allergies. There is hope for millions of people plagued by severe allergies throughout the globe as the future seems to be one of ongoing discovery and advancement.

www.ingramcontent.com/pod-product-compliance
Lightning Source LLC
Chambersburg PA
CBHW050814250726

48653CB00006B/2226